Organising health events for women

Organising health events for women

Edited by Hazel Slavin
From material by Marie Armitage, Carol Beaumont, Liz Hall,
Janice Marks, Linda Pepper, Jan Smithies, Mary Tidyman

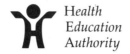
Health Education Authority

Published in 1991

Health Education Authority
Hamilton House
Mabledon Place
London WC1H 9TX

© Health Education Authority 1991

ISBN 1 85448 236 X

Printed in England by Belmont Press

Contents

Foreword
Introduction   1

Key issues   3
  Diversity   3
  Childcare   5
  Content   8
  Summary   10

Planning and finance   11
  Why and what?   11
  Who?   13
  When and where?   15
  How?   16
  Finance   18
  Summary   24

Publicity   25
  Publicity leaflet   25
  Booking form   28
  Pre-event materials   29
  Press coverage and advertising   32
  Summary   34

Running the event   35
  Choosing the venue   35
  Establishing the climate   37
  Central information services   38
  Speakers and facilitators   41

Social events	42
Ending	44
Summary	45

Evaluation 47
   Methods 47
   Collecting data 48
   Summary 51

Checklists 52
Planning 52
Publicity and materials 52
Organisation of event 53
Afterwards 54

Appendices
Appendix 1: Running workshops 55
Appendix 2: Resources 57
Appendix 3: Useful addresses 58

Acknowledgements 60

Foreword

The Health Education Authority is a special Health Authority within the National Health Service. The general principles guiding the HEA's approach to health education include working in partnership with other organisations and individuals, and fostering creativity and enterprise in health education so as to encourage self-confidence and self-reliance.

The HEA is committed to taking account of the special needs of a number of groups, including those of women. The HEA's Field Development Division has responsibility for the coordination of work relating to women's health. It is concerned with enabling key health workers and others to enhance their skills and abilities to undertake effective health education using a range of appropriate approaches, whatever the changing patterns of health and disease.

This booklet is based on the experience of planning and running the National Women's Health Conference in Liverpool in July 1989, which was funded by the HEA. It offers guidelines and models of good practice which we hope will be useful for anyone organising a health event for women.

Introduction

This booklet is for women, both professional and lay, working in the statutory and voluntary sectors or in the community, who want to run health events for women. It provides advice and checklists to help in the planning, running and evaluation of conferences and workshops. It has its roots in the National Women's Health Conference 'Feeling Strong, Growing Stronger' held in Liverpool in July 1989. It provides a record of the conference by using the experiences of the women who organised and participated in the event. Throughout the booklet you will find highlighted text like that below. This indicates that it has been based directly on the experiences of planning and running the conference held in Liverpool, and illuminates the reality of working and planning together.

As a planning group we came together with excitement and a vision of what a conference organised by women for women might be. We had very different levels of experience in organising events and varied personal and professional reasons for getting involved. As individuals and as a group of women working collectively for the first time we grew and developed throughout the planning process and the conference itself. For several months afterwards we continued to meet to evaluate, share and write up our experiences and those of other women, of the event itself and the process involved.

The booklet is designed in sections which contain information followed by a summary of 'things to remember'. You will also find a set of checklists at the end of the booklet which you can photocopy and use to check your planning progress.

You can, of course, use any or all of the sections you need, but you are strongly advised to read the section on 'Key issues' whatever the size of the event you are running.

Key issues

This section focuses on three key issues that need to be considered from the outset. These are:

- Diversity
- Childcare
- Content

Diversity

Your health event is likely to be for:

- women from black and ethnic minorities
- women with disabilities
- women from different classes
- women of different ages
- women with differing sexualities
- women with differing childcare needs

The issue of diversity is central in planning as well as running events. It is important that women working in the area of women's health are from a wide variety of backgrounds, races, ages, abilities and environments and that they have different priorities, needs and ways of working. Differences between women are potentially very positive and provide a wide range of ideas and ways from which we can all learn.

The challenge is to be able to work together where possible, acknowledging that differences include elements of power imbalance and oppression, for example between black and white women. Clearly this can cause major barriers which make working together difficult and it is important that these issues are not glossed over. As well as differences between women there are similarities which require identification so that work can be undertaken in a coordinated way.

When organising events it is important to be aware of differences and to try and involve a range of women from the beginning. However, it is wrong to assume, for example, that having several black women, lesbians, or women with disabilities in a group means that this is enough in itself. It will provide a perspective but not all the views of black women, lesbians or women with disabilities (an impossible task). Furthermore, these women should not be expected to take total responsibility for ensuring that attempts are made to meet the needs of lesbians, black women, or women with disabilities. They should not have their involvement in a project or event limited to their experience of race, sexuality or ability. It must be recognised that it is sometimes difficult to involve some women because they face financial or time constraints.

What is needed is a strategy from the outset about how all oppressions are going to be handled during the planning process and the event itself. It may be worth drawing on the experiences of other women's groups by inviting them for discussions or by reading and sharing views or articles about, for example, black and white women working together.

There are lots of contradictory issues about differences, which is why it is so challenging and very stimulating and why it can create new openings and directions. Remember though that many women do not neatly fit into categories, indeed some may fit into several: for example, a woman may be older and black, disabled and a lesbian. This is an issue to bear in mind when trying to provide separate space for women to meet.

The lesson here is to continue to offer separate space as part of the main agenda but to try and avoid clashes where women are forced to choose between different parts of themselves. Another option is to leave space within the timetable for women to set up their own specific workshops or meetings, although this may be interpreted as the organisers failing to take responsibility.

Whichever way a conference or event is structured, whether around workshops and/or interest groups, all groups should consider difference and oppression. This aim needs to be made clear to both facilitators and participants.

Childcare

Without crèche provision many women would not be able to attend a women's health event. Indeed, the prospect of high quality childcare might attract women to events where all too often childcare is a secondary, rather than a primary, consideration.

Your planning group needs to consider:

- who will organise the crèche?
- who will work in it?
- do they need training?
- what equipment will they need?
- where should the crèche be?
- will you use male crèche workers?
- how will you get information about the children (number, ages)?
- will the crèche run all day and all evening?
- financial issues

Organisation

It was agreed that we employ someone with experience to take on responsibility for the organisation of the crèche and that all crèche workers would take part in a training day which would highlight the requirements of anti-sexist, anti-racist and multi-cultural crèche provision. The training day would also give those workers who had not previously worked together the opportunity to develop a system of co-working for the conference weekend.

Thirty-four crèche workers were identified. We did not know how many children would come to the conference so we decided to pay all crèche workers a fee if they were not needed. Those who attended the training day were also paid.

Important considerations

■ From the onset of planning an event there needs to be close liaison between the planning group and the crèche coordinators.

■ If the event is likely to have large numbers of children or a wide range of ages, it may be necessary to have separate coordinators for different age groups.

■ It is helpful to employ crèche workers of different cultural backgrounds, at least to reflect the mix of women at the event.

■ Childcare is of primary importance and paying the going rate for the job, at least Nursery Nurse Examination Board rates, goes some way to recognising it as such.

■ Crèche workers need regular breaks for tea/coffee and meals, so cover may need to be organised to allow for this.

■ Rooms allocated for a crèche should be checked

prior to the event for safety and suitability. They should be away from meeting rooms because of noise, but near enough to allow time for settling and collecting children.

■ Budgeting for a crèche may need to include costs for workers, hire of equipment including cots, highchairs and play resources, taxi fares for babysitters. Money should be available at least two weeks before the event to allow materials to be purchased or deposits paid.

■ The crèche should offer a good experience for the children by including interesting activities as well as the opportunity to meet children from other areas and backgrounds.

■ All crèche workers should have police clearance to work with children. This is routine with people who work with children.

■ Women may be offered a choice of whether or not to allow male workers to care for their child/ren.

■ In order to organise a good crèche, it is necessary to know how many children will need childcare as early as possible – ideally, one month before the event.

Arrangements

The crèche was provided from 9 a.m. to 9.15 p.m. We also provided a babysitting service on Friday between 7.15 p.m. and 11 p.m. and on Saturday from 7.15 p.m. to midnight. This was arranged so that women could put their children to bed and attend evening events without worry. Babysitters were paid to 'listen in' on each landing once children had been put to bed.

There was a room for under-fives and another, larger room for over-fives. A range of suitable activities were offered, including play-doh, sand and water, paints, table-top equipment, craft activities, games and songs, and a trip to a local museum and across the Mersey.

Content

There is a variety of ways of organising the content of an event. You might choose to have a selection of:

- interest groups
- topic groups
- lectures and speakers
- workshops
- leisure events
- events purely for fun

Interest groups are for groups of women with specific concerns. You might offer the opportunity for women to meet separately with other women with whom they especially identify. This might be because of race, class, sexuality or another identifying and unifying feature.

Topic groups allow groups of women to meet to learn and talk about a specific health topic such as 'healthy eating', 'inequalities in access to clinics' or 'positive cervical smear tests'. Topics chosen will be related to the aims and objectives of the event.

Lectures and speakers can motivate women and are useful for imparting information or putting across a point of view. However, make sure the event doesn't consist solely of lectures and speakers. You need also to provide the opportunity for women to talk and learn together in a structured way.

Workshops provide structured and facilitated time for learning and sharing. They provide an opportunity for every woman to speak and listen. They must have clear aims and objectives and facilitators should be thoroughly briefed.

Leisure events are useful for dividing the time at a longer event. Organising leisure events linked to health in particular serves the dual functions of introducing women to new techniques and 'keeping healthy' strategies as well as providing time to be sociable. You could think about providing sessions such as massage, aromatherapy, swimming, drama and dance or stress and relaxation.

> *Sessions planned were banner making, homeopathy/ allergies, massage and aromatherapy, circle dance, voice, self-defence, stretch to music, cooperative games and crafts, stress and relaxation, creative writing, drama and photography/video.*
>
> *As well as the sessions originally planned, an unexpected trip to the local sports centre was offered. Rather conveniently for the conference, the centre was holding a special 'Into Sport' day which had many new and unusual sports on offer, including scuba diving, free of charge, for people wanting to try them out for the first time. Some women went along to this session and returned enthusiastic and delighted with their achievements.*

Events purely for fun allow organisers to be creative: parties, discos, picnics, special 'theme' evenings can raise morale as well as provide the opportunity for women to meet informally.

> *We aimed to make the weekend as enjoyable and memorable as possible for the women attending. Social events were seen as an integral part of the event.*
>
> *We planned circle dancing and had the bar available following speakers on Friday night for a relaxed and soothing atmosphere. On Saturday night Women and Theatre and Tacktlass performed followed by a disco – a more lively and celebratory occasion.*

Summary: Key issues

Diversity

Difference is positive
Plan for inclusion not exclusion
Be aware of difference
Ensure a diverse planning group

Childcare

Is childcare to be provided?
Who will run the crèche?
Will it run throughout the event?
Will workers need training?
What equipment is needed?

Content

Will the event be topic-based?
Will it have speakers or lecturers?
Will it be workshop-based?
Can it provide leisure events?
Will it have social time?

Planning and finance

This section is to help you plan your health event. It looks at:

- Why and what?
- Who?
- When and where?
- How?
- Finance

Why and what?

> Early ideas for a National Women's Health Conference emerged from discussions between workers in Merseyside and an officer at the Health Education Authority

The earliest stages of planning and fund raising can raise difficulties. This is because it may be necessary to provide a rationale and aims and objectives in order to get funding. It is, however, unrealistic to expect that detailed planning can take place before funding is secured. Planning takes time and money. Early discussions must be tentative because if funding isn't agreed there may be a problem about raising expectations which can't be met.

Aims and objectives

The first important task of a planning group is to set realistic aims and objectives. The aim is the overall intention of your event. It is not specific, it is what you hope to do in a general way.

AIM
To bring together women, both unpaid and paid, who are actively involved in the provision of health education and health care for women in their community.

You achieve your aim by breaking it down into objectives. The objectives of the event are specific, measurable, achievable, realistic and time-related. You use your objectives to evaluate and keep you on target when planning and running the event.

OBJECTIVES

- *To create a positive, stimulating and lively atmosphere to support exchange of ideas and dialogue.*

- *To ensure participation from a representative group of women and in particular to reflect cultural diversity.*

- *To enable active participation of these diverse groups in all aspects of the conference, including planning and organisation.*

- *To develop a model of good practice' for conference organisation that focuses on the process of enabling participation in all aspects of the conference for all women.*

- *To raise awareness about women's health education and practice.*

- *To develop tactics and strategies which integrate women's particular needs in all aspects of health education and care.*

Who?

Who an event is for is intimately bound up with the aims and objectives. The event may be for professionals, a mixture of professional and lay women, or for any woman who is interested in health issues. The planning group must be clear about target groups, and the content and publicity should reflect the audience.

AIM
To bring together women, both unpaid and paid, who are actively involved in the provision of health education and health care in their community.

The publicity said:

WOMEN'S HEALTH GROUPS all over Britain are actively involved in providing informal health education and health care for women. These organisations vary according to the needs of the local area, from an informal health information drop-in, or a support group on a housing estate, to a Well Woman Centre offering a comprehensive service, including a listening ear, information and medical screening tests. What all the groups have in common is their concept of health as being 'a state of complete physical, mental and emotional well-being, and not just the absence of disease' (World Health Organization definition). They also recognise that social and economic factors can affect women's prospects of achieving good health, e.g. poverty, racism, age, lack of transport, lack of good childcare, poor housing, etc.

But the reality was:

By initially aiming the conference at only women's health groups there was a danger of identifying health

> *too narrowly. For example, black women organise in ways which are most appropriate to themselves and their community. Often when they discuss or organise around health issues and related concerns, they may not be in groups which call themselves 'health groups'.*

The planning group must be clear about who the event is for. It might be a health event for black women, for women living in rural areas, for lesbians, for professionals working with other women, for women working with voluntary groups. It is important for the publicity to reflect this and for the content to be relevant.

> *The planning group was committed to trying to ensure that the conference was open to a wide range of women with a particular priority for black and ethnic minority women, women with disabilities, women involved in unpaid voluntary and community work, rural women and working class women.*

It is not enough to say that the event is, for example, for black women without black women being part of the entire process of planning, organising and evaluating the event. It is easy to alienate individuals and groups with good intentions. This can be seen as patronising and tokenistic.

> *A crisis was reached in terms of recognising the problems around lack of involvement of black women. The black planning group member did not attend a two-day meeting and subsequently left the planning group. There had been other challenges at local meetings about the lack of involvement of black women. As a group of white women, it was difficult to be confronted with our own racism and to respond to that criticism, particularly given time constraints. The planning group considered carefully whether the conference should go ahead, bearing in mind its original aims of ensuring participation from a representative*

group of women, in particular to reflect cultural diversity, and to enable active participation of these groups in all aspects of the conference, including planning and organisation. The group decided to go ahead with the conference providing a number of strategies were pursued to tackle the issue:

■ *the local conference organiser would prioritise outreach work with black women in Liverpool in order to explain about the conference and encourage participation*

■ *input would be encouraged from black women at national level, including the HEA and Black Health Forum*

■ *there would be a concerted attempt to ensure that the issues and needs of black women's health were an integral and central element to the organisation and agenda of the whole conference*

■ *a full contribution from black women to the conference would be sought by attempting to ensure that a high proportion of interest group facilitators, speakers, workshop facilitators, crèche workers and others were black*

When and where?

There are a number of issues to consider when planning the timing of an event. The funding may determine when an event is held, for example, sometimes money has to be spent before the end of the financial year. The timing of other events, national and local, may affect your decision about when to hold your event. It is important to remember that you will need time to plan and organise. It is important to be realistic about what needs to be done. It may take up to two years to plan and mount a national event.

Liverpool was seen as a very suitable venue for a national conference as it was already the site of a great deal of creative and innovative women's health work with the involvement of many paid and unpaid women who could contribute a great deal to conference planning.

Remember:

■ avoid term times if you want to use university or polytechnic halls of residence

■ avoid arranging your event too near holidays, such as religious festivals or bank holidays

■ check local and national publicity to see whether the dates for your event clash with anything similar, or conflicting

■ school holidays may be the best, or worst, time for your event depending on your target group and will have implications for childcare arrangements

■ check that the venue is easily accessible by public transport

■ check that the venue is accessible for women with disabilities

How?

Whatever your event is to be, it is essential to set up a planning group in good time. Remember that it may take up to two years to mount a national event, and perhaps six months to organise a one-day or half-day event properly. In setting up a planning group you need to consider:

■ which groups need representation

■ how to ensure a balance between what is practical and achievable and what is wanted by different groups with differing perspectives

■ whether you need a representative from a national organisation

- when and how the group meets
- whether the group needs a 'team building' event
- where the funding for planning will be found
- whether specific tasks of planning and organisation will be allocated to individuals or small groups

It is important to note that the planning group were not experts, but were a group of women with different experiences and skills, all of whom learnt an enormous amount through the process of planning this conference. One of the many things that we learnt was the extent to which other women perceived us, at least before the conference, as a remote, faceless planning group. The collective responsibility of the group was an important element of the planning process and was a real strength of the group, as was demonstrated through the way in which members supported each other, shared tasks, and took joint decisions around the challenges.

Specific tasks might be allocated. These could include:

- finding and securing venue
- finance
- childcare arrangements
- food
- finding and briefing facilitators
- publicity
- dealing with local/national media
- social events
- administration before, during and after the event
- organising, writing and printing materials

- registration, chairing and welcoming duties
- organising displays

How many times the planning group meets will be determined partly by the size of the event. The important thing is to set up your planning group early enough to plan efficiently and thoroughly.

Finance

The main source of funding for the Women's Health Conference was the Health Education Authority. In autumn 1988 a proposal for funding a National Women's Health Conference was approved by the HEA. At this time very little detail about the conference had been developed, so it was difficult to gauge the amount of money required.

To make informed estimates of costs you will need to consider:

- **Pre-event costs**
    - meetings: travel and subsistence
    - publicity
    - administrative support
    - stationery, postage and telephone
    - organisers' time
- **Event costs**
    - venue and food
    - travel
    - childcare
    - payment for facilitators/speakers
    - bursaries for attendance
    - social events
    - equipment

■ **After-event costs**
- de-briefing meeting
- evaluation reports
- report of event
- administrative tasks such as 'thank you' letters

You should then consider how you might raise income:

■ **Income**
- grants
- sponsorship
- attendance fees
- money-raising events such as a bar or bookstall

Raising income

Sponsorship

Some organisations will provide services such as photocopying, or free use of venue instead of providing cash.

> Additional funding was obtained from other sources. Two Liverpool charities, the Eleanor Rathbone Trust and the John Moores Foundation, contributed funds for bursaries for local women to attend the conference. Free use of some local facilities was offered to conference participants by the city council (an example of payment in kind).
> The Save the Children Fund contributed £200 towards the cost of childcare at the conference.
> The Scottish Health Education Group, the Health Promotion Authority for Wales, and the Northern Ireland Health Promotion Unit each sponsored some places for women from those countries to attend. Clwyd NALGO and the Clwyd Health Authority both sponsored two local women to attend.

> There was not enough time to seek commercial sponsorship for the event.

Obtaining sponsorship for an event requires very early planning. You may need to apply for sponsorship at least one year ahead of the event.

Remember though that sponsorship may be controversial and the planning team will need to establish criteria to decide whether sponsors are acceptable or not.

Fees for attendance

> The planning group was committed to trying to ensure that the conference was open to a wide range of women, with a particular priority for black and ethnic minority women, women with disabilities, women involved in unpaid voluntary and community work, rural women and working class women. It was essential to be able to offer a substantial amount of money in the form of bursaries to allow the targeted women to attend.
>
> Financial assistance was offered in a number of ways:
> - assistance with travel expenses
> - waiver of part or all of conference fees
> - free accommodation in local homes

It is possible to have two rates of fee: one for women who are sponsored by their workplace or other organisation and a second, lower rate for women paying for themselves.

If your event hasn't got a sponsorship or grant 'cushion' it is essential to cost it carefully and charge fees which will cover the costs. Always add a percentage (about 15 per cent) for unforeseen costs. Remember you could always return money if there's some left over, but you won't be able to ask for more once you have set your fee, so you could end up making a loss.

Who is paid?

Early decisions need to be made about who is to be paid. It is unusual to pay a fee to a planning group, but not for the planning group to hire someone, on a short-term contract, to be the event organiser. Obviously, this is only relevant for events such as residential conferences.

Some events are funded well enough to pay a substantial fee to workshop facilitators and lecturers. Other events ask for facilitators to work for no fee and simply provide expenses.

Many women contributed to the planning and organising of the conference, the training of women to work at the conference, and the running of workshops, interest groups, 'Look After Yourself' sessions, social events and other elements of the conference. Some did this as part of their usual paid work, although often contributing many hours over and above what they were paid for. Some were paid from the conference budget to undertake a specific task, for example the crèche coordinators, the crèche workers, women performing at the social event. Other women were unpaid and volunteered their time, being reimbursed for any expenses incurred. For example, seven women were invited to give a short presentation during the opening session of the conference. They were given their travel expenses and overnight accommodation.

The funding for the conference was not large enough to enable payments to be made to all the women involved and a number of issues were considered when deciding about who could or would be paid. For example, would paying facilitators make their contribution seem more valuable than that of other participants?

Some other financial tips

Before and during the event there will be a need for cash. For example, it may be necessary to equip a crèche with a first-aid kit, disposable nappies and other consumables. Crèche workers (and baby-sitters) will need to be paid. Stationery and other miscellaneous items will need to be bought such as blu-tack, flip chart paper, badges, pens and so on. Some women may need money in advance to travel to the event.

■ It may be easier to raise money for 'capital' ('one-off') items such as equipment, printing or hire of premises. 'On-going' or 'revenue' budgets involving the cost of salaries may be more difficult to fund.

■ There are some key sources for funding, such as:
- statutory agencies such as health authorities, local authorities, community health councils
- trusts and charities
- commercial companies
- fund raising activities
- trades unions

■ It may be possible to fund raise locally for particular initiatives in support of the event. Some members of the planning group could take responsibility for this.

■ Budget enough for planning group expenses, especially if the event is a national one. Travel costs can be substantial, and if you are building them into your budget, remember to allow for inflation costs.

■ If a training event for facilitators and planners is held before your event, some women will lose income and may have to be reimbursed.

■ Check with women that a payment does not affect their state benefits.

■ Women need to be informed in good time if they are to be given financial help to attend the event.

■ Using free accommodation in local homes is a good way of reducing costs, but takes a lot of time to organise. Some women will not feel at ease with this idea and it may be intimidating for them. Women who are not residential at a 'residential' conference may well miss out on the important social and 'fringe' events.

■ It helps to have someone on the planning group who takes the responsibility for organising the financial matters.

Summary: Planning and finance

Planning

Why a women's health event?
What is the aim?
What are the objectives?
Who is the event for?
Where will it be held?
When will it be held?
How will the planning group ensure balance and representation?

Funding

Pre-event costs
Event costs
After event costs
Raising income
- sponsorship
- grants
- attendance fees

Who is paid?
Other financial tips
- make sure you have cash available
- try raising money for capital expenses
- try all the key sources for funding
- try fund raising locally
- budget for planning group expenses

Publicity

Good, well-targeted publicity is very important if the event is to be well-attended. This section looks at:

- the publicity leaflet
- the booking form
- pre-event materials
- press coverage and advertising

The planning group needs to make an early decision about how to attract women to the event. There are a number of ways of advertising an event, including publicity leaflets, press coverage and advertising through local or national media, and pre-event material.

Publicity leaflet: design, content and scheduling

The publicity needs to be sent out well in advance of the event to ensure as wide a distribution as possible, and also to allow time to gather as much information as possible about participants' needs in terms of access, childcare, translators, bursaries, special dietary needs and so on.
The publicity for the event needs to include:

- the aims and objectives
- the venue
- the dates

- the purpose of the event
- special statements if required

If possible use the work of a professional to design material for your event. Keep the design simple and striking. Don't try to include too much information: this will come in the form of a pre-event pack.

> As we were very well-funded for this event (by women's health work standards) we were able to use a professional designer to produce the leaflet. [See opposite] We chose a woman who had already designed for another national women's event and whose work addressed multi-cultural images of women, and used colour in a creative way. The design included fairly abstract images that did not indicate age, class, race, etc. The publicity style was very well received by women and gave the conference a lively image from the outset.

If you are organising a big event it may be helpful to have a logo to help establish an identity. The logo can be used on all material and on signs and badges at the event.

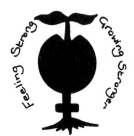

National Conference for Women's Health Groups

Distribution

> We aimed to distribute the leaflet through a wide range of health education and women's networks and organisations. In all we produced 4,000 copies of the leaflet – and achieved our target number of 200 partici-

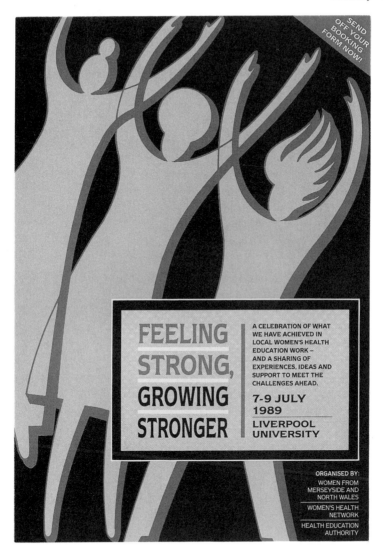

pants. We also targeted black health networks, though subsequently we learnt of other possible mailings, contacts and networks. Five hundred leaflets went to Liverpool for local distribution, and the rest were sent out through a variety of networks and mailings.

The section on useful addresses at the end of this booklet contains the addresses of organisations which can help with publicity. The usual arrangement is for that organisation to include your publicity leaflet with their mailing. Some agencies only mail at certain times of the year, so it's important to have your publicity ready early.

Booking form: content and design

The form which is returned to the organisers needs to include:

- name, address, telephone number
- special requirements (food, access, signing, translating)
- details of childcare required
- application for a bursary or waiving of fees
- personal details in case you have to prioritise places
- Positive Action Statement (see opposite)

The form should, if possible, reflect the design style of the publicity leaflet - in terms of colour, logo, typeface, etc.

Pre-event materials

Participants will need:

- a letter confirming their place at the event
- programme
- venue address and map

POSITIVE ACTION STATEMENT

The conference organisers are committed to trying to ensure that this national event is open to a wide range of women. A number of places are reserved for women from Merseyside and Deeside. By reserving some places for women from Scotland, Northern Ireland and Wales we are particularly hoping that they will travel and meet with women from England at the conference.

It is hoped that all women who apply will be able to attend.

If, however, applications **exceed 200** the following will be taken into account:

• involving women from organisations rather than individuals • no more than two women from each group • a fair regional spread of participants • a mix of different ages:

Please indicate which of the following you consider yourself to be:

☐ Young   ☐ Middle   ☐ Older

Within the above, women who are part of the following groups will be given priority. Please tick any you consider to include you:

☐ Black or ethnic minority   ☐ Rural
☐ Disabled   ☐ Working class
☐ Unpaid/voluntary/community

(The above information will only be used for the purpose stated and will remain confidential.)

BOOKING A PLACE

Please tick one:

☐ Enclosed is a cheque/PO for £ _____
(payable to *Health Education Authority*)

☐ Please invoice _____

_____

for the sum of £ _____

Return this completed booking form to our Conference booking agents:

Rosemary McMahon, Andrea Donsey
Professional Briefings
189a Old Brompton Road
London SW5 0AR

Tel: 071-370 4437

■■■■■■■ **CLOSING DATE: 9 JUNE 1989** ■■■■■■■

■ information about lectures, workshops and other sessions
■ information about leisure, social and fun events
■ local travel information
■ information about childcare

30 Organising health events for women

The planning group will need to devise a form to be returned if there is a choice of options. This form should give information on:

- what childcare is needed
- what sort of accommodation is needed
- if there are special mobility or dietary requirements

An example of the pre-conference form for the crèche can be seen on the next page.

Below is another example of how to collect information: women have to make a choice for an 'interest' group:

| INTEREST GROUPS | There will be three sessions during the conference at which women will join **one** interest group to look at: |

Session 1 – Introductions, and work women have done so far
Session 2 – Evaluating work individually and collectively
Session 3 – What women need to do to meet the challenges ahead

Please indicate your first **three** choices of interest groups below, **in order of preference**. *(Except in exceptional circumstances, interest groups will not run if less than 10 women opt to join them.)*

☐ Black women

☐ Asian women ☐ Well women centres

☐ Minority ethnic women ☐ Community/voluntary groups

☐ Unwaged/unemployed women ☐ Women with disabilities

☐ Working class women ☐ Women with children

☐ Older women ☐ Health information, education and resources

☐ Young women ☐ General (mix or range of women at the conference)

☐ Fat women

Pre-conference form

"Feeling Strong, Growing Stronger"
Liverpool University, 7-9 July 1989

CRÈCHE FORM

Please fill in a form for each child you are bringing to the conference, and return it immediately in the stamped addressed envelope provided.

CHILD'S NAME: ....

    SEX: ....

    AGE: ....

ANY SPECIAL NEEDS/DISABILITIES/ALLERGIES?   YES/NO
(Please specify)

....

....

SPECIAL FOOD REQUIREMENTS (including food children **definitely** will not eat):

....

PLEASE TICK IF YOU

☐ DO NEED A TRAVEL COT
☐ DO *NOT* NEED COT BEDDING

PLEASE INDICATE ANY SPECIAL REQUIREMENTS CONCERNING SLEEPING ARRANGEMENTS:

....

IF ENGLISH IS NOT YOUR CHILD'S FIRST LANGUAGE, DOES SHE/HE NEED SOMEONE WITH THEM TO HELP WITH LANGUAGE?

                                                                         YES/NO

IF YES, WHICH LANGUAGE? ....

PLEASE TICK THIS BOX IF YOU DO NOT WISH YOUR CHILD TO BE LOOKED AFTER BY A MALE CRÈCHE WORKER ☐

I AGREE TO MY CHILD GOING ON THE ORGANISED OUTING   YES/NO

NAME .... SIGNATURE ....

Thank you for completing this form – Please return urgently in the enclosed S.A.E.

Some things to remember

There are conflicting pulls on publicity. Firstly, the need to advertise the event as widely and as far in advance as possible; and secondly the need to include as much material and information as possible, so that women are clear about what exactly they are booking for. There are two rounds of publicity: the first drawing women's attention to the event in general terms, and the second containing more detailed information and a booking form. In a large scale event with a wide range of different needs, women should book their places at least six weeks before the event to allow the planning group to respond effectively to their various requests. This means final publicity and booking forms should be distributed at least three months before the event.

■ It may be worth pre-testing your publicity material to see if the language, tone, content and images used are acceptable to all women.

■ It is important to use clear language to indicate who the event is for, or to make clear who an event is particularly aimed at. There will always be women who have different views and who find certain language or labels offensive. Be clear and be sensitive.

■ There will be a need to publicise the event to far more women than actually attend. Make use of mailing lists and contacts or your publicity will not reach the women you are targeting for the event.

Press coverage and advertising

■ Press coverage is much easier to obtain at a local level, on the whole, than at a national level. The press are looking for a newsworthy story, and this needs to be borne in mind when writing a press release. Different emphasis may be needed for local and national press. Linking the event to something else that is currently newsworthy is also a good tactic.

■ Try to get as much free publicity as possible through the press or radio, but take great care that the event is not misrepresented. Send clear press releases and ask to see articles or hear radio interviews before they go out.

■ During the event it is useful to have one or two women specifically available to deal with the media. The press and local radio need chasing before, during and immediately after the event for coverage, and this takes a lot of time and effort at a time when there are other immediate and pressing practical tasks to be done.

Summary: Publicity

Who will write and design publicity material?
Does the event need a logo?
Who is the target audience?
What information is put out?
- date
- time
- place
- some content details
- price

When should material be ready?
What information is required from participants?
- childcare
- special dietary needs
- mobility requirements

What distribution lists are available for publicity?
What do you need for pre-event materials?
- letter of confirmation
- programme
- venue address and map
- information about lectures, workshops and other sessions
- information about leisure, social and fun events
- local travel information
- information about childcare

Running the event

Of course, every planning group will run events differently, but there are some considerations that will set you well on your way to running the event smoothly. These are:

- choosing the venue
- establishing the climate
- having central information services
- properly briefing speakers, lecturers and facilitators
- holding social events
- ending positively

Choosing the venue

These are some of the things the planning group will have to consider when choosing a venue:

- cost
- a pleasant environment
- easy access by rail, bus and car
- access for women with disabilities
- residential accommodation if appropriate
- meeting rooms
- rooms suitable for workshops and social events

- suitable accommodation for crèche
- catering facilities to provide for a variety of diets

University and polytechnic halls of residence can be reasonably cheap to hire and often have good facilities for meetings and workshops. Another advantage of using this type of accommodation is that the staff are used to event delegates and are usually able to help with any problems. Special conference centres are usually more expensive and less easily accessible by public transport. However, they are often situated in pleasant surroundings and they have the advantage of being 'one-sited' – meeting rooms are usually in the same building as bedrooms. This may not be the case with university or polytechnic accommodation where quite long walks may be involved.

Some hotels offer good rates for conference events. They usually quote a 'conference package' whether the event is a half-day or two or three days. Look carefully at the details of the package. Some include meeting rooms, audio-visual equipment and flip charts, while others make an extra charge.

Catering is often a source of complaint.

> We wanted to ensure that the kitchen staff could provide food suitable for vegetarians, children, any cultural or religious diets requested and particular health diets if necessary (for example, for women who were diabetic or had coeliac disease). Bread and milk was available in the accommodation blocks to make bed-time snacks for children.

Remember that the planning group will need the information about special dietary needs well in advance of the event, so that catering staff can be alerted and make the necessary arrangements.

If your event is going to be accessible to women with disabilities, the planning group will need to check that the accommodation is suitable.

- Is there ground floor accommodation?
- Are there ramps for wheelchairs?
- Are there toilets nearby for women with continence problems?
- Are there lifts as well as stairs for those who have mobility or fitness problems?

Other considerations:

- accessibility for prams and buggies
- whether disabled women bring a carer
- quiet space for breast feeding mothers
- special facilities for women who are blind
- signing arrangements for women who are deaf
- loop system for women with partial hearing

> *We underestimated the amount of stair climbing involved throughout the weekend! Because of tight timetabling and the need to change rooms between workshops, interest groups, coffee and meal breaks, etc. women often had to rush up and down stairs. Some women became tired, others had difficulty breathing, one facilitator had a fear of heights to overcome. This added to their stress and caused delays.*

Establishing the climate

It is important to try to create an environment to meet the needs of women attending the event. The planning team needs to ensure that as far as possible it can provide:

- a friendly and supportive atmosphere

- a way for women to express their practical needs and to be able to meet them
- a flexible and efficient organisation to respond to changing needs
- a forum for effective communication
- opportunities for women to meet socially
- a mechanism for participants to feel that they are part of the event and can influence its direction
- a non-oppressive atmosphere

> The aims were always ambitious and could never have been totally met. Some of them, like the 'atmosphere', were the responsibility of those attending as well as the planning group.
>
> The care and concern provided that weekend was unique in the lives of some women attending. They became absorbed in the excitement and debate.
>
> Some decisions we made were wrong – the most obvious one being the temptation to cram too much into two days. More time was needed to allow 200 women to get up and down stairs to sessions, coffee etc, collect children from the crèche and settle them again after meal times and to find which room they were supposed to be in at any given time! This undermined the intended relaxing atmosphere.

Central information services

> We were aware that the registration desk is often the first contact women have with the conference and we wanted it to be welcoming, organised and not pressured – as first impressions can set the tone of the event.

Organisers, and that usually means the planning group, need to arrive at the venue well in advance of the participants to establish a registration desk. Try and make the registration area uncluttered and welcoming. The registration desk needs to have spare copies of all pre-event materials for participants who either didn't receive them or have forgotten to bring them.

For residential events, where participants have travelled some distance, workers on the registration desk need to be prepared to deal with some tired, hungry and anxious women and children. Smiling and being welcoming isn't easy to sustain, so share out the task of working on the desk.

Ensure you have:

- clear signposting
- the crèche open
- maps of the venue if necessary
- enough copies of materials and hand-outs
- refreshments

This is what we gave to participants on their arrival:

WELCOME

Welcome to the Women's Health Conference. We hope this conference will provide a positive and stimulating environment for women to meet, share information and discuss the strengths and weaknesses of work on women's health and the challenges which face us in the future.

The full participation of all women at this conference is vital for its success. Because of this we would like all of us to be aware that we come from different backgrounds and that we may have different needs and ways of working.

Language or behaviour which stereotypes, discriminates against or insults all women or particular groups of women, e.g. black women, ethnic minority women,

> lesbians, working class women, older women, is not acceptable and will undermine the conference.
>
> If such problems arise attempts should be made to address them. The planning group will assist in this process if women wish.
>
> Please feel free to talk to us on this or any other matter (including problems with conference organisation).

If you are organising a two-day (or longer) event, it is worth establishing an 'events office' as this will be the focal point for information and communication. Ideally, it should be equipped with a telephone and photocopier. Organisers will be inundated with information requests.

The conference office provided information on:

- taxi numbers
- local places of interest
- local maps
- railway and bus timetables
- places of worship
- doctors, hospitals, chemists
- first aiders
- off licences
- restaurants and takeaways with their various prices
- nearest shops, like newsagents and the post office
- local sports centre opening times

It is useful to have an 'event box' too, even for a half-day event. This box should contain a variety of useful things such as:

- post-it notes
- stapler
- paper clips
- felt-tip markers
- paper
- pens
- flip charts
- pencils
- rubbers
- sellotape
- spare bulb for OHP
- screwdriver
- extension lead
- first aid box
- sanitary towels and tampons

Speakers and facilitators

Speakers and facilitators must be properly briefed about how and where the session for which they are responsible fits into the overall event. A member of the planning group should speak with each facilitator or speaker and explain the aims and objectives of the event and any special features. It is also useful to follow this up with a clear, written brief.

If your event has a number of speakers who will be talking to many of the participants, it is important to aim for a running order to provide for a variety of style and subject. Less experienced speakers usually prefer to go first but don't assume that experienced speakers won't be nervous! Provide water for speakers and try to minimise problems by checking microphones and audio-visual equipment and organising the room so that everyone can see and hear.

> We planned to have seven speakers on the Friday evening. These would be representative of different women involved in women's health, such as older women, black women, women from different parts of the UK and international speakers. We would also have presentations on racism, the White Paper on the NHS Review and the Women's Health Network. It was planned as a very informal session. Each speaker was to talk for 15 minutes followed by questions and general discussion.
>
> Women who agreed to facilitate workshops were sent written information about what was expected, the times of workshop sessions and forms to indicate which sessions they would prefer or were available for, and what resources such as videos or overhead projectors they required. Workshop facilitators (and interest group facilitators) were sent guidelines of key issues identified by the planning group for encouraging an open environment while being aware of oppressive behaviour.

If possible, arrange for speakers and facilitators to meet before the event begins and give them a tour of the venue and facilities.

> There was a briefing session held for workshop facilitators on the Friday prior to the opening session. The material sent out to facilitators was discussed, questions were answered, and time and room allocations were explained.

Social events

Social events are important at events which last more than

one day. They should be relevant to the theme of the event and as carefully planned as other parts of the event.

The planning group needs to:

- liaise with performers
- decide whether alcohol will be available
- negotiate for women bar staff
- ensure that plenty of non-alcoholic drinks are available
- decide if the social events are open to women who are not attending the event
- find out if music or alcohol licences are needed
- pay performers
- allow for impromptu participation
- organise who will be responsible for clearing up

> The theatre group and women's band on Saturday night were excellent. A local woman DJ organised music. The evening was an emotional release for many women after the difficult issues of the day. Women were determined to enjoy themselves and did so. Some danced until the early hours and then went for a walk or continued socialising.
>
> The children enjoyed themselves and at one point staged a takeover of the sound system. There were also impromptu contributions from women who had attended a voice workshop.
>
> There were some problems however. Some of the Asian women did not join the social because alcohol was being sold. Negotiations were needed with the porters and security staff to allow dancing to go on late.

Ending

It is important for any event, however long or short, to have a recognisable ending. This can be linked with evaluation and can be an opportunity for participants to say what they feel about their experiences. Plenary sessions can be tedious if they only consist of 'reporting back', and the emotional temperature of the occasion can sink too low for participants to go away feeling positive. To make sure your event finishes on a positive note:

- allow time for verbal feedback
- encourage participants to say goodbye to each other
- allow for the release of emotion

> *The closing session was planned to take place in the large meeting room with women being asked to fill in two post-it stickers saying:*
> *– What I am leaving behind at the conference*
> *– What I am taking away with me*
> *The planning group decided to invite criticism and suggestions but not to attempt to answer them at the time. Many women came to the microphone – some confidently, others nervously, wanting to share their comments and feelings about the conference.*

Make sure you take care of practical considerations:

- allow time to clear up
- remind everyone to return questionnaires and evaluation forms if you are using them
- check train times and adjust your closing session to meet these
- identify lost property

The planning group too needs to have an ending or debriefing session.

Summary: Running the event

Choosing the venue

- cost
- pleasant environment
- easy access by public transport
- meeting rooms
- amount and type of residential accommodation
- room for crèche
- catering facilities

Establishing the climate

- a friendly and supportive atmosphere
- a forum for communication
- opportunity for women to meet socially
- a mechanism for participants to feel they are part of the event and can influence its direction
- a non-oppressive atmosphere

Central information services

- effective and welcoming registration desk
- event office
- event box

Properly briefing speakers and facilitators

- well-planned running order
- check technical equipment works

Holding social events

■ make sure these are relevant to event and appeal to all participants

Ending positively

■ allow time for verbal feedback

■ allow for the release of emotion

■ make sure you have taken practicalities like train times into consideration

Evaluation

Evaluation is often seen either as a daunting chore to be done at the end of an event to satisfy the funders or as an academic exercise requiring precise statistical skills. Viewed more positively, creative evaluation can be a way of finding out what went well – and less well – so that the planning group and others can learn from the experience. This section looks briefly at how this can be done effectively. It looks at:

- methods
- evaluation forms
- group and individual evaluation

Methods

Events can be evaluated by examining the **process** and the **outcome**, by using methods which are **qualitative** and **quantitative.**

The planning team must consider the purpose of any evaluation, decide who it is for, who will do it and disseminate the findings as well as information about the methods used.

Qualitative methods are those which supply answers to questions (i.e. feelings, ideas, opinions); quantitative methods use numbers as their basis (i.e. *how many* participants enjoyed the opening session etc.) Ideally the evaluation should start at the planning stages of the event and both methods should be used to record and assess the process.

The *process* can be evaluated by recording the planning and implementation of the event.

Methods of doing this include:

- diary keeping
- questionnaires
- individual interviews
- group interviews

Similar methods can be used during the event. Participants can assess the venue, atmosphere, content and social aspects, as well as determine whether they feel the health event has achieved the objectives set by the planning group (the *outcome*).

Collecting data

Evaluation forms can be imaginatively designed to collect both quantitative and qualitative data. Participants may find it more satisfactory to be given their evaluation forms at the beginning of the event, so they can fill them in during the proceedings. Try to use a variety of methods and assessment techniques:

- ask direct questions:
'Was objective 3 met?'

- ask open-ended questions:
'How did you feel about having to choose two workshops from a list of five?'

- use rating scales:
'Rate the food on this scale: 0 = poor ——— 10 = excellent'

- collect numbers:
'How many sessions did you attend?'

■ collect comments:
'What did you most enjoy?'
'What would you like to say to the planning group?'

> An evaluation sheet – with open-ended, wide-ranging questions – was distributed to all women during the last few hours of the conference. Women were asked to complete the form and leave it at the information desk before they left.
> A total of 59 completed questionnaires was returned. Most of these were given in at the end of the conference, although some trickled in later, having been sent to individual women on the planning group. This return was disappointing. Having a return address at the bottom of the evaluation sheet may have resulted in more being returned – many women are in a hurry to get away at the end of an event and are more likely to fill in an evaluation sheet later if it is obvious where to send it!

Group evaluation can be a rich way to evaluate within an ethos of participative working.

■ small groups can fill flip chart paper with comments

■ groups can discuss how they felt about the event and present this to others

■ groups can negotiate a 'group answer' to a set of questions

Participants can make an individual evaluation which can be presented to everyone.

> 'Post-it' stickers were used at the closing session of the conference. Women were asked to write 'one thing I am leaving behind at the conference' on one sticker and 'one thing I am taking away from the conference' on another. These were displayed for everyone to see.

The planning group will need to evaluate whether or not the event achieved its objectives.

The booking forms provided valuable information on the geographical areas women lived in, their age range, whether they were paid workers or voluntary, disabled, from rural areas, from black or ethnic minority groups, and whether they considered themselves working class. This information helped us to evaluate whether or not our aim of attracting specific groups of women had been achieved.

One surprising finding of our analysis was that while many participants perceived low numbers of black and ethnic minority women attending, the booking forms revealed that almost 25 per cent of participants defined themselves as being from ethnic minority groups.

Summary: Evaluation

Evaluation methods

qualitative (answers to questions)
quantitative (numbers)

Evaluate

process (what happened)
outcome (did the event meet its objectives)

Collecting data

diaries
questionnaires
individual interviews
group interviews
counting
rating scales
public announcements
ending games
negotiated group statements
analysis of booking forms

Checklists

Use these checklists to make sure you have covered everything.

Planning   *See pages*

Planning group identified	3–4, 14, 16–17	☐
Dates organised	15–16	☐
Rationale agreed	11	☐
Aims set	12	☐
Objectives set	12	☐
Venue booked	15, 16, 35–37	☐
Sponsorship: National	19–20, 22	☐
Local		
Industry		
Voluntary Sector		
Other		
Fee set	18–19, 20	☐
Finance organisation allocated	23	☐
Evaluation methods chosen	47–50	☐

Publicity and materials

Designer appointed	26	☐
Leaflet written	25–26, 32	☐
Poster written	25–26, 32	☐
Logo agreed	26	☐
Mailing lists compiled	26, 28, 32	☐

Mailing addresses identified 28 ☐
Local media contacted 32–33 ☐
National media contacted 32–33 ☐
Pre-event materials written 28–32 ☐
Pre-event materials printed 32 ☐
Displays organised 18 ☐
Maps ready 29 ☐

Organisation of event

Child care	crèche organiser appointed	5–6	☐
	crèche venue agreed	6–7	☐
	crèche workers identified	6–7	☐
	training identified	6	☐
	cost to participants agreed	7, 18–19	☐
	first aid box organised	22	☐
	consumables bought	7, 22	☐
	cash for crèche workers available	7, 22	☐
	babysitting service organised	7	☐
	payment for babysitting ready	7, 22	☐
Venue:	venue visited	16, 17	☐
	catering staff briefed	36	☐
	disabled access identified	36–37	☐
	notices and signs made	38–39	☐
Event:	keynote speaker(s)	8, 41–42	☐
	lecturers	8, 41–42	☐
	workshop facilitators	8, 41–42	☐
	interest groups	4–5, 8	☐
	topic groups	4–5, 8	☐
	free time identified	9	☐
	social events identified	9, 42–43	☐
	bar organised	19, 43	☐
	leisure facilities identified	40	☐
	chairing duties arranged	18	☐
	registration desk organised	18, 38–40	☐

event box established 40 ☐
event office organised 40 ☐
ending session planned 44 ☐

Afterwards

venue account settled 23 ☐
expenses paid 22–23, 43 ☐
thank you letters written — ☐
planning group de-briefed 44 ☐
evaluation report written 47–50 ☐
accounts closed 23 ☐

Appendix 1: Running workshops

It is likely that any health event will include some time for participants to get together in workshops. The major principles of this type of work are:

- starting from where women are
- using the knowledge and experience of participants

The facilitator is responsible for:

- the physical space
- the objectives of the session
- introductions and climate building
- structuring the time
- managing the process
- participating in evaluation

The physical space needs to support a learning environment where participants can contribute their knowledge, feelings and experience. Ideally, everyone should sit in a circle or horseshoe in comfortable chairs that can be moved to form pairs or small groups. Sometimes workshops are held in less than ideal situations, but at the very least the facilitator should ensure that everyone can see and hear each other.

The facilitator's role includes setting the goals of the session although, of course, these can be refined and negotiated by the participants. One of the objectives might be 'to set realistic targets for the workshop' or 'get to know each other better'. The facilitator must provide:

- a structure for this to take place

■ a working climate which encourages the fullest participation.

These principles are important whether the workshop is to share knowledge and information, feelings (support groups) or debate issues and share experiences.

A structure for a 2½ hour workshop might include:

■ a brief introduction from the facilitator
■ a name game and 'getting to know you' exercise
■ agreeing some ground rules for the group
■ agreeing purpose and objectives
■ structured exercises (the work of the group)
■ a review of work
■ a review of process (if relevant)
■ ending and evaluation

Appendix 2 : Resources

Measuring Change, Making Changes: An Approach to Evaluation. Lois Graessle and Sue Kingsley, 1986. London Community Health Resource.
No Time for Women: A Workbook for Discussion Groups. Charmian Kenner, 1985. Pandora Press.
Greater Expectations: A Source Book for Working with Girls and Young Women. Tricia Szirom and Sue Dyson, 1986. (British edition edited: Hazel Slavin). Wisbech Learning Development Aids.
Women and Health: Activities and Materials for use in Women's Health Courses and Discussion Groups. 1987. Health Education Council/Workers Education Association.
Working with Groups. Antoinette Satow and Martin Evans, 1983. HEA/TACADE.
Working Together. Bryce Taylor 1983. Oasis Publications.
Graphics Handbook: An Introduction to Design and Printing for the Non-specialist. Richard McCann, 1985. HEC/NEC.

Appendix 3: Useful addresses

Black Health Forum
c/o National Community
Health Resource
57 Chalton Street
London NW1 1HU

Brook Advisory Centre
153a East Street
London SE17 2SD

DAWN
Drugs, Alcohol, Women Now
Omnibus Workspace
39–41 North Road
Islington, London N7 1FT

Equal Opportunities Commission
Overseas House
Quay Street
Manchester M3 3HN

Family Planning Association
27–35 Mortimer Street
London W1N 7RJ

Fawcett Library
City of London Polytechnic
Old Castle Street
London E1 7NY

Feminist Archive
Bath University
Claverton Down
Bath BA2 7AY

Health Education Authority
Hamilton House
Mabledon Place
London WC1H 9TX

Health Education Authority's Assertiveness and Women's Health Project
c/o Health Education Authority
Field Development Division
Hamilton House
Mabledon Place
London WC1H 9TX

Health Education Authority's Health Education for Women Training Project
c/o Health Education Authority
Field Development Division
Hamilton House
Mabledon Place
London WC1H 9TX

Health Promotional Authority for Wales
8th Floor, Brunel House
2 Fitzalan Road
Cardiff CF2 1EB

Lesbian Line
BM Box 1514
London C1N 3XX

London Black Women's Health Action Project
Bethnal Green Hospital
Cambridge Heath Road
London E2 9NP

National Abortion Campaign
75 Kingsway
London WC2

National Community Health Resource
57 Chalton Street
London NW1 1HU

Northern Ireland Health Promotion Agency
The Beeches
12 Hampton Manor Drive
Belfast BT7 3EN

Oasis Publications
Beechwood Conference Centre
Elmete Lane
Leeds LS8 2LQ

Scottish Health Education Group
Woodburn House
Canaan Lane
Edinburgh EH10 4SG

Sheba Feminist Publishers
48 Kingsland Road
London E8 4AE

Sickle Cell Society
Greenlodge
Barretts Green Road
London NW10 7AP

The Women's Press Ltd
34 Great Sutton Street
London EC1 0DX

Women's Educational Advisory Committee
Workers Education Association
9 Upper Berkeley Street
London W1H 8BY

Women's Health Forum
Health Education Authority
Hamilton House
Mabledon Place
London WC1H 9TX

Women's Health Network
National Community Health Resource
57 Chalton Street
London NW1 1HU

Women's Health and Reproductive Rights Information Centre
WHRRIC
52 Featherstone Street
London EC1Y 8RT

Women's National Cancer Control Campaign
1 South Audley Street
London W1Y 5DQ

Women's Therapy Centre
6 Manor Gardens
London N7 6LA

Acknowledgements

We would like to thank all the people and organisations who contributed in so many ways to the National Women's Health Conference, Liverpool, July 1989:

Crèche coordinators: Cheryl Williams and Maureen Waygood
Crèche workers
Women in Merseyside involved in local planning:
    Sheila Gregory, for organising billeting
    Leigh Stevens, for organising food
National Community Health Resource (NCHR):
    Training project workers: Sara Hill and Monica Knight
    Other workers: Jane Lethbridge, Fiona Kearns, Paula McDiarmid, Sarah Underwood, Roland Dovan and Peter Watson

Health Education Authority staff: Bina Patel, Caroline Coulter and Sally Atkinson.
For funding and sponsorship:
    The Health Education Authority (Professional & Community Development Division and AIDS Division)
    Eleanor Rathbone Trust, Liverpool
    John Moores Foundation, Liverpool
    Save the Children Fund
    Scottish Health Education Group
    Health Promotion Authority Wales
    Northern Ireland Health Promotion Unit
    Other organisations who sponsored individual women to attend the conference

For the loan of crèche equipment:
    The Gregson Playgroup, Merseyside

Acknowledgements

Merseyside Trade Union Resource Centre, Children's Centre
Wirral Under Five's Centre

Jenny Heywood from The Glenda Jackson Theatre
Staff at Liverpool University Derby and Rathbone Halls of Residence.
Professional Briefings for administrative support
Family Planning Association, Liverpool
Liverpool (Central & Southern) Community Health Council
Community Relations Council, Liverpool
Liverpool Black Sisters
Interest group facilitators, training - Georgina Webster & Irma Phillips
Interest group facilitators
Workshop facilitators
Look After Yourself session facilitators

Speakers:
    Carol Beaumont, Women's Health Network
    Lucy Billagera, Nicaragua
    Zelda Curtis, Older Women's Network
    Kathleen Feenan, Women's Education Project, Belfast
    Edel Teague, Women's Education Project, Belfast
    Linda Pepper, Health Education for Women Training Project
    Margueritte Woods, Ana Liffey Project, Dublin

Social organisers: Caroline Marsh and Nicky Crosby
Performers at the social
    TACTLASS, from Sheffield
    Women in Theatre, Birmingham
    Monica Knight
    Gerry Rowlands, circle dance

Lee Robinson, for designing the publicity leaflet
News from Nowhere, Women's Cooperative Bookshop, Liverpool
Margaret Citrine, Disablement Resource Unit, Liverpool for advising on disabled access
Planning group members:

Marie Armitage, Wirral Women's Health Network
Carol Beaumont, Women's Health Network
Jan Gill, Wirral Women's Health Network (up to May 1989)
Liz Hall, Local Conference Organiser
Janice Marks, Delyn Community Agency, Clwyd
Linda Pepper, Health Education for Women Training Project
Pauline Caddick, Community Relations Council Liverpool
Liverpool Black Sisters (up to May 1989)
Jan Smithies, Health Education Authority, Community Development
Pat Thorney, Women's Health Information Support Centre, Liverpool (up to June 1989)
Mary Tidyman, Health Education Authority, Women's Health Education Coordinator

And last, but by no means least, all the women who came and contributed in so many ways to the weekend, and the children for enriching the weekend.